The Beautiful Language of the Heart
Where evolution is inviting us to go

ANAMIKA

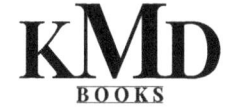

KMD
BOOKS

Copyright © Anamika Neitlich

First published in Australia in 2024
by KMD Books
Waikiki, WA 6169

All rights reserved. No part of this book may be used or reproduced by any means, graphic, electronic, or mechanical, including photocopying, recording, taping or by any information storage retrieval system without the written permission of the copyright owner except in the case of brief quotations embodied in critical articles and reviews.

Because of the dynamic nature of the Internet, any web addresses or links contained in this book may have changed since publication and may no longer be vaild. The views expressed in this work are solely those of the author and do not necessarily reflect the views of the publisher and the publisher hereby disclaims any responsibility for them.

Typeset in Adobe Garamond Pro 12.5/18pt

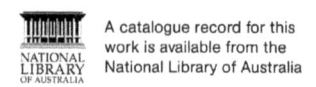

A catalogue record for this work is available from the National Library of Australia

National Library of Australia Catalogue-in-Publication data:

The Beautiful Language of the Heart/Anamika

ISBN: 978-1-7636194-4-9
(Hardback)

Contents

Foreword 1
Introduction 3
Chapter 1: The Human Journey 7
Chapter 2: Isolation 14
Chapter 3: I'm Broken 19
Chapter 4: Survival Fears 26
Chapter 5: Feeling All Feelings 35
Chapter 6: Experiencing Ourselves 41
Chapter 7: Starting to Accept Himself 46
Chapter 8: Feeling Connected 52
Chapter 9: Gentle and Forgiving 60
Chapter 10: Self-Love 66
Chapter 11: Understanding Life 71
About the Author 87
Introducing The Beautiful Language of the Heart Documentary .. 88

Foreword

I've always been interested in understanding more about myself, but I simply had no idea of the shadow until I met Anamika. Working with her helped me tame the untamed chaos of my mind.

As for the shadow … JM Barrie knew about this and sewed it to the foot of Peter Pan … Lewis Carroll took Alice down the rabbit hole of the mind, and so we learn and grow.

Food was my comfort. I used food to try and cope with pain I didn't yet know how to handle. Then came Anamika. She helped me heal, calm my mind, and be more kind to myself.

When Anamika showed me the documentary she made about her work with Vaughn Dorn, who has non-speaking autism, I was so moved. It helped me understand so much more about not only my shadow and its limited beliefs, but how to experience my real self.

There is a world of the unknown in each of us that can be brought to light. With Vaughn, Anamika dove in to help him feel it, see it, and express it so that we can experience it too.

Vaughn's story is unique and inspiring. It is an example to the world of what's possible in finding yourself… so don't give up on anyone and don't give up on yourself.

Although Vaughn has autism, this book is not only about autism. It's about the human journey itself; the journey that Vaughn is on, the journey that I'm on, and the journey that each of us travels in our own way.

Vaughn is so eloquent. Like many others, sometimes I express myself so clumsily, my words getting in a muddle. But what is not in a muddle is my passion for this journey. It's what I care so much about!

This book will shine a light on your inner world, like it did on mine. It reaches into the heart and soul to reveal larger truths and life-changing revelations.

Read on dear readers, read on.

– Sarah Ferguson, Duchess of York

Introduction

Twenty-six years ago, I received an unexpected and surprising phone call. A distinctly British female voice was on the other end. "Hello, it was suggested that I contact you for healing and guidance. This is Sarah Ferguson, the Duchess of York, by the way."

I spontaneously drew a deep breath, not because of who I was talking to, but from the magnificence of what I felt. I was instantly moved by the beauty of her heart and soul, beyond all of the layers of her personality and her title, as she was reaching for help to find her real self.

Four years ago, I received another unexpected and surprising phone call. A female voice calling from California pleaded, "Can you help my son Vaughn? He's twenty years old, has autism and doesn't speak, but he can communicate with you by typing."

"I'm so sorry, but as much as I'd like to help, I have no experience with autism," I responded. Beth insisted, "You don't need any experience. Just do what you do to reach him so he can express his thoughts and feelings. Help him come out of his shell and find himself."

The first time I sat with Vaughn on Zoom, I spontaneously drew a deep breath. His unfiltered authenticity and emotional availability moved me to tears. There was such simple richness in connecting with each other as we sat together in silence. I could feel the expansive beauty of his heart and soul, deeper than his personality, beyond his autism, reaching to connect, reaching to know his real self.

Though living very different lives, Sarah and Vaughn were both in pain. They had both experienced feeling isolated, misunderstood, harshly judged, and bullied. They wanted to heal, understand themselves, and find peace and self-love.

When I showed Sarah the documentary I had made of my sessions with Vaughn called *The Beautiful Language of the Heart*, tears came to her eyes. "You and Vaughn have helped me understand so much more about myself. His is a unique story and I believe it will give courage and hope to people globally."

This book and its companion documentary chronicle the journey of finding oneself, as seen through the eyes of an extraordinary young man. We accompany Vaughn as he emerges from crushing isolation, expresses his pain, discovers his unique gifts and purpose, and finds joy in being the amazing person that he is. He learns to communicate beyond words with the beautiful language of the heart.

Sharing Vaughn's inspirational transformation from pain to joy allows insight into making that same shift more deeply in our own life. This is particularly relevant for each of us now during this time of great change, as the world is becoming new.

There's so much pain in the world, yet it was never meant

The Beautiful Language of the Heart

to be that way. Unexpressed pain accumulates and obscures the abundance of love that's available. When we express our pain we heal, and the beauty of our light shines through.

It's where evolution
is
inviting us
to go.

We're at a time in human evolution that's inviting us to heal our pain and surrender our sense of separateness. It's inviting us to experience connections in which we feel seen, heard, and safe. It's inviting us to hold ourselves and each other in tender acceptance, forgiveness, and compassion. It's inviting us to open our hearts and live from our innate desire to feel, express, and share love.

Evolution is inviting us
to explore
beyond
what we think
we already know.

We're being invited to become not only who we've always dreamed we could be, but so much more that it's unimaginable. We're invited to touch the awe-inspiring beauty of our multi-dimensional nature, which is not based on our thoughts, our words, or how we think things are. Who we are is so much deeper and more expansive. In these limitless dimensions, we can touch the mystery, magic and joy of life.

In these energies, there are ways of communicating that are not solely based on language. They are instantaneous and richer than what language alone can provide. When we feel the energy of who we are beyond words, in the depths of our being, from the reaches of our soul and spirit, and from our oneness with All That Is, we are speaking the beautiful language of the heart.

Thank you for joining us on this journey. Most of all, thank you for the willingness, courage and self-love it takes to explore new perspectives, to fulfill the promise you made to yourself to come home to the magnificent person you truly are, and to keep becoming more.

With my love,
Anamika

Chapter 1
The Human Journey

*We wish to be free of bondage
and the suffering it causes.
We yearn for something
beyond the ordinary.*

When I first met Vaughn, he was in a lot of pain. He had been dealing with intense challenges with non-speaking autism since he was very young. I got to know his story little by little through our weekly sessions on Zoom, which have been ongoing for three years to date.

Before introducing you to Vaughn and his story, let's set the stage by understanding his journey within a larger context. There's something monumental happening in the world during this current era that's impacting my journey, your journey and Vaughn's journey.

Each era is a dream that dies as a new one is being born. In any era, the strongest matrix of ideas becomes a paradigm. It's a pattern that creates what we call reality. This pattern takes on a life of its own and becomes an operating system. It's the "box" in which we live, and whose edges constrain our thinking.

There have been different paradigms on our planet. One paradigm shift occurred when people went from thinking the Earth was flat to the Earth was round. These days, round seems normal, but a change in perspective such as from flat to round causes a shift in the whole paradigm that is the norm in that era.

In our present era, we are also going through a paradigm shift, but this one doesn't have to do with the shape of the Earth. It has to do with the shape of human consciousness itself, which metaphorically is going from flat to round. Each of us is personally invited to embrace that shift, as is the whole of humanity.

Every paradigm has its own underlying perceptions that we take for granted as real or "reality" because we grew up thinking they were normal. We're not usually aware of these underlying perspectives and beliefs, and most people don't necessarily question what they think is real; it just seems like the way things are.

A change in perspective affects everything and turns our way of seeing inside out and upside down. It's a gradual process because the change in a paradigm takes time to be fully accepted. It doesn't come without a lot of opposition to the new perspective. While change is exciting, it can also elicit fear and dread, which take time to move through.

We're in that period during our evolutionary process in which our current fear-based paradigm is crumbling along with the birthing of something new. The turmoil happening throughout the world is part of the collapse of the old paradigm, precisely

The Beautiful Language of the Heart

because we're in the process of changing perspectives. It's not an indication of something going wrong, but of evolution.

Right now, the magnitude of change in the world is so great it's almost incomprehensible. We've reached the extremes of our current way of thinking, being and relating. It's no longer working, and we are outgrowing it collectively as well as personally. We're living through the death rattle of an old order that is collapsing on itself. When it reaches its edges, it implodes and consumes itself. We are at those edges now.

Living through the dismantling can be challenging. It's easy to feel confused, angry, scared and helpless. It can bring up deep issues in each of us that are ready to heal. Even though it might look like the world is going insane, falling apart, or even coming to an end, what is occurring is not the end of the world. It's the end of what doesn't work.

Regardless of how ugly and disturbing it can feel on the planet right now, or how bleak and terrible the future might seem, the world isn't being destroyed. As scary as it can be to live through the tragedy, pain and crises that so many people are experiencing, now is the time for life-changing breakthroughs and rebirth for each of us personally as well as collectively.

The hatred and insanity of separation, divisiveness, domination and control that are inherent in flat consciousness are being exposed at a level as never before. Although it can be difficult to witness and live through, we can't heal something until we're aware that it's there.

As the current fear-based paradigm collapses, a new, round love-based, grace-filled cooperative consciousness is being born. Now, more than ever, we can grow beyond the traumatized, hurt, and disconnected places within us that don't feel safe and loved. In this new expanded consciousness we feel safe, connected, loved, understood, nourished, free, peaceful, joyous, and so much more.

Flat to round

This change in perspective from separation to connection is supported by discoveries in quantum physics. The fact that we're not separate, but are all interconnected, changes everything. It changes how we feel, how we relate, how we live, and how and what we create. It also changes what we're able to see and experience.

You might wonder if humanity is going to survive the collapse, violence and breakdown that's happening. We will indeed! Our planet and humanity are evolving beautifully. We have already decided that we will succeed. A new future full of hope, born of our light, and filled with an alive vitality is already emerging.

What's happening in the world is also happening inside of each of us. Evolution is inviting each of us to a radical change in our individual consciousness from flat to round. We don't need to be in pain to change.

We can willingly choose to participate in this seismic shift so that we personally can live joyously in the present.

As much as our spirit loves change, we can resist when we're afraid that the accompanying chaos will be ominous. But chaos can be healthy, and can open us into the magic and mystery of what is not yet known.

The Beautiful Language of the Heart

*We're in the process
of our world becoming new
and
chaos
accompanies
change.*

Despite the enormous suffering that still exists in our world, we've already crossed the midline into birthing a brighter future. Becoming more acutely aware of our personal and collective darkness born of separation, is part of this evolutionary change. Collectively, we're learning what it means to be compassionate, inclusive, and interconnected human beings.

*Humanity is yearning
for the experience
of knowing ourselves
as one world
and
as part of a greater whole.
We long to feel ourselves
as one with All That Is
as a tangible embodied experience.
We can sense that who we are is
greater than what we have ever known
and we came here to experience that greater self.*

As much as we might want to grow and change, it takes courage to keep opening beyond our resistance into the uncharted territory of a new self and a new life we haven't yet experienced. When we are willing to stretch beyond who we think we are and beyond whatever we think we know, we ignite sparks of new life.

The perception within flat consciousness is that we are not only separate from each other, but from our multidimensional self and from All That Is. Even though we live in a three-dimensional world, we are not only three-dimensional beings. We are actually multidimensional. Our consciousness is infinite and expands so far beyond our third dimensional reality that it's impossible for the linear mind to comprehend.

This means that each of us is not an isolated "I" separate from a larger whole. We are interconnected through resonance fields of energy in which we are still our own personal selves and are also connected in oneness at the same time. This is the paradox of both/and which the linear mind doesn't understand because it thinks in either/or.

Flat to round

When we embrace paradox and truly experience ourselves as interconnected and part of a greater whole, we're never alone or without support and resources. We can open to receive what we need rather than trying to shoulder everything ourselves. We can value all that exists and treat ourselves and each other with dignity, love, and respect.

Even though humanity as a whole still lives within a survival perspective to a large degree, and it takes time to evolve beyond it, we individually can go ahead to explore and discover what is humanly possible. As we personally evolve, we have an enormous

The Beautiful Language of the Heart

impact on helping humanity evolve, because our new, round consciousness effortlessly radiates its joyous positivity.

This paradigm shift in our consciousness is a true metamorphosis. A caterpillar, in its metamorphosis, is transformed into a whole new being following a total dissolution of its previous form.

A butterfly is not
a caterpillar with wings.

We, too, are becoming something new, something greater than we were, far beyond who we've been, beyond what we've dreamed, and beyond our ability to imagine. And new really means new; it has never existed before!

Chapter 2
Isolation

I got to know Vaughn's story through our weekly sessions on Zoom. His parents, Beth and Ryan, told me that signs of autism appeared early in his life after he was already a physically coordinated toddler who was speaking a few words. When autism set in, he lost his speech, auditory processing, and ease of physical movement.

At age seven, he learned to type letter by letter with one finger. Despite years of professional help that assisted him to develop his brain in certain ways, something was still missing. He lived within a shell of isolation. Even though he could type, he didn't know how to communicate his thoughts and feelings. He couldn't break out of his shell.

Vaughn's mom Beth reached out to me because of my years of experience connecting with others nonverbally through energy, as well as verbally. In our first session, I didn't ask Vaughn to come out of his shell. I sat in silence and connected with him underneath and beyond his autism. My energy reached him,

The Beautiful Language of the Heart

which let him know that he wasn't alone.

He could feel me being present with him right away. I was in awe of how exquisitely attuned and profoundly aware he was, how beautifully transparent with no filters. He let me in right away as he could feel me accepting and appreciating him exactly as he was. Without any words passing between us, he could tell that I wasn't judging him, so he began to open up. He typed that he was so relieved to finally be communicating because he had lived in crushing isolation his whole life, feeling broken, and trapped in a body that he couldn't control.

I let him know that I understood his anger and frustration. I also saw what a highly sensitive and extremely loving person he was, who was frightened to come out of his shell. His trust had been broken after so many years of rejection because of his autism. "Vaughn, I don't define you by your autism. To me, you are you, a beautiful being first and foremost."

He looked at me a bit confused and amazed. He was used to being judged, misunderstood, and rejected. Other than his very caring family, most people didn't take the time to get to know him. As a result, he had become numb from rejection, making it difficult for him to take in my words. He couldn't believe he was being understood.

The more he felt me being truly present with him, he became more hopeful and communicative. Each week, he would share more nonverbally with his energy, body language, facial expressions, sounds, and by typing. Gradually, he started to come out of his shell and move toward his deepest desires to express, connect, and love.

I let him know that his face and body were extremely

expressive and he was communicating with his energy brilliantly without realizing it. He thought he was not communicating, when in fact he was, and always had been.

It's very easy to understand why Vaughn would feel isolated given the particular challenges of his autism. Again, while never comparing one person's life with another, we all have experiences of feeling isolated for different reasons. We've all experienced feeling alone, misunderstood, not heard, and as if we don't matter.

Basic human nature wants to love, to feel alive, to express, and to create. Everyone craves feeling met, loved, understood and connected. To deny our most basic and inherent desires causes terrible suffering and pain. It causes anger, frustration, hopelessness, and desperate attempts to escape the pain.

As Vaughn and I sat together, he got to experience the feeling of connection he had been seeking. I felt the profundity of our connection as well. It was palpable and full of love. As he softened and surrendered into that connection, he began to feel the dynamic flow of his own energy moving through his body, between us, and all around him.

Feeling our true flow
alters our reality
uplifting us
into realms of the miraculous.

He also began to see the judgmental beliefs he was harboring about himself. It was these beliefs that were keeping him in isolation, blocking him from being open to the love and connection he craved the most.

The Beautiful Language of the Heart

I let him know that staying guarded and defended is painfully isolating, even though at certain stages of life it might have been necessary. Armor is an energy block, a hardened, contracted state. It's a prison of loneliness in which we deny ourselves love even while yearning for it.

When we keep our defenses in place, it diminishes our impact. As we retreat, withdraw, hide, or pull away, revealing less of who we are, we experience less, and have less impact. In withdrawal, we can be quite numb. This kind of separation from ourselves is extremely painful and greatly reduces our impact.

Fortunately, we can open up. I assured him that being open is not a dangerous place to be, although it can feel scary as we open up. Open heartedness is not passivity, nor vulnerability that leaves us available for further hurt. It's a vibrant, active state in which we experience ourselves as safe and loved in our connection with All That Is. Then, we don't need to put up walls of protection because we naturally have healthy boundaries. There's nothing to protect or defend against since we are connected with All That Is through love.

However, just declaring we are open does not let down the armor and open the heart. Opening begins by gently focusing within our heart and becoming non-judgmentally aware of the armor. As we meet our armor with acceptance that it's there, it will express its resistance and then gradually relax. It can sometimes be accompanied by tears, which like rain, soften the hardened ground.

*Defenses dissolve
into an ocean of tenderness.*

Anamika

In these warm waves of energy
we feel loved
safe
and
home.

Chapter 3

I'm Broken

Vaughn was interested in exploring the negative beliefs that made up his defensive armor. He was convinced that it was his autism and lack of speech that were causing his isolation and pain. He was sure that there was something wrong with him.

When I asked him what he thought was wrong with him, he stated with no hesitation and with great certainty, "I'm broken and need fixing." It hurt my heart that he felt that way about himself, because it's so clear that he's a whole and wonderful person as he is.

On the other hand, I understood him feeling that way because everyone feels not good enough in some ways. I looked him right in the eye and said, "Vaughn, there is nothing wrong with you, including your autism. You are whole and wonderful exactly as you are. So let's talk about self-judgment, ok?"

He looked interested in what I had to say, but was not yet on board with changing his mind. He was so sure he was right about how broken he was.

"I understand that you think there's something wrong with you because you don't speak. When we judge ourselves, we're basically saying that we're unacceptable as we are; we're not good enough. When judgments become extreme, we can hate ourselves, want to get rid of certain parts of us, or even want to die. The harshness of judging ourselves creates pain in our emotional and physical bodies."

As a result of his negative self-judgments, Vaughn could see that he was suffering terribly. He felt trapped, because he thought that if he fixed the autism he would feel better, but he couldn't fix the autism. "It can seem that your suffering is coming from your circumstances. Your autism certainly presents challenges, but since you can't change your autism right this second, and it also has great gifts to offer you, let's experiment with changing your point of view."

Based on his past experiences of being judged and feeling there was something wrong with him, Vaughn had retreated into an inner vault of isolation to feel safe. He had erected barriers for defense and protection and remained defended in his vault. He was perpetually on guard, waiting for the next criticism. He got so used to judgment that when it wasn't coming from someone else, he continued to perpetrate it upon himself with his daily refrain, "I'm broken and need fixing."

When we live behind barriers, we wonder why we're isolated, impoverished, unhappy, unhealthy, and unsuccessful. We can feel alone even when we're with other people and not understand why. We can have millions of dollars and never feel like it's enough. We can take good care of ourselves and do all the "right" things, but still not feel well.

The Beautiful Language of the Heart

Vaughn was starting to see that the beliefs he harbored about himself had formed mental loops that were depressing. He could feel their weight and pressure in his head, chest and whole body. "I never realized that these beliefs were so heavy and were weighing me down. They feel like cement barriers."

Barriers are impenetrable.
They armor our heart and
shut down our luscious flow of energy.
They block the aliveness
and
joy of life.

As Vaughn began to recognize that his barriers were there, and understand why he constructed them, he began the gentle un-defending of his heart.

Barriers are not boundaries
and
boundaries are not barriers.

Healthy boundaries are like a permeable cell membrane. They allow the cell to maintain its distinct identity while receiving life-giving nutrients. I asked him to imagine himself as one cell within a loving body that is protecting and nourishing him. "Now how do you feel?" I inquired. He closed his eyes to contemplate for a moment, then typed excitedly, "I feel safe! There's no need for walls of defense, or barriers. There's nothing to protect against."

"Yes, and that's how our relationship is with All That Is. When we feel connected instead of alone behind our barriers, we feel safe as part of a loving whole." He sat back and closed his eyes as he was taking this in. We sat in the stillness together. When he finally opened his eyes, a relaxed and peaceful Vaughn was there.

His next question was to find out how to do this on his own the next time he started beating himself up about being broken. First, I reassured him that none of this was his fault. It's very easy for everyone to get seduced by our fear-based self-judgments. When we believe what they tell us, we can get overwhelmed by the pain those judgments cause.

These fear-based beliefs come from our primitive brain. Its orientation is, "What do I have to do to save myself or to fix this or that? How can I get more? How can I be in control of my life? What do I have to do to get somewhere?" It thinks it's solely responsible for everything, like a little cell with no bigger body nourishing it. It's in a constant panic, feeling responsible for its own survival. It doesn't realize it can relax and receive from the bigger body.

Vaughn gradually saw that his suffering was actually coming from the negative stories and judgments he made up about himself, which he then believed. We made a list of his most repetitive stories or beliefs so that he could start to recognize them as they recycled. This helped him realize that he didn't have to keep believing them, no matter how real they seemed in the moment.

His list was just like that of many other people: "There's something wrong with me, I'm not safe, my life is hopeless, I need to try harder, I need to be better than I am, I should be perfect, I'm not enough, I'm not lovable, I'm not of value, I have no impact, I don't matter, other people will judge me and never take the time to get to know me."

In thinking he should be different than he was, he kept holding himself to some false sense of perfection that he could never meet. Then he would get mad at himself and frustrated with his life. He discovered that the bad feelings he kept having were predominantly coming from his self-judgments and limiting beliefs, rather than from his circumstances.

He was learning to accept whatever the current limitations of his autism were, and to find the gifts in it, which were plentiful. He could begin to feel the dignity that comes from accepting himself exactly as he is in each moment. When he rejected himself, he didn't experience that he was already abundantly lovable, capable and wise just as he was.

*Through acceptance
of who we are
and where we are
in this present moment,
growth and change
happen naturally.*

He could easily tell the difference between how bad the judgments feel in his body and how good acceptance feels. His anxiety, depression, and pressure came from his mental checklist of unrealistic demands he kept putting on himself to hurry up and fix himself.

These bottomless demands went on all day in his mind because within the world of "never good enough" nothing ever seems good enough, most especially us. Even when we meet our goals, we're still never good enough. Like a donkey chasing a carrot that's always out in front, the donkey never gets the carrot. When we continue to chase a carrot that we fail to catch, it produces a cycle of suffering in which we get:

Frustrated, impatient
anxious, desperate, afraid,
stressed, strained
clenched, tense
depleted, exhausted
discouraged, depressed.
Sick, pressured
humiliated, blamed, shamed
outraged, in-raged
hostile, rejecting, rebellious
vengeful, vindictive
self-pitying, punishing
resentful.
Powerless and hopeless.
Utterly separate, completely alone.
Insular, isolated.
Collapsed.
Numb
despairing,
apathetic,
wanting to die.
We pick ourselves up.
Try harder.

The Beautiful Language of the Heart

Fight harder.
Work longer, go faster, do more.
Spike adrenaline.
Push, dominate, demand.
Consume, possess.
It's still not working.
Complain, plead, submit, give up.
We're in crisis.
This is the cycle of suffering.

Fortunately, we can get beyond our judgments because they are not actually real, no matter how real they might seem. Negative judgment is completely different than healthy discernment and acceptance of our limitations as well as gifts. When we regard our judgments simply as fear stories, no matter how real they might feel, and boldly choose a more empowering perspective, we feel liberated and free.

"Vaughn, when you negatively judge yourself and then try to pressure and force yourself to be different, you feel hopeless and despairing. By accepting yourself as you are in this moment, you can feel good about yourself even with your current limitations.

"When we feel good, there's positive motivation to make the changes we can. Through acceptance, some of your limitations may actually change, and whether or not they do, you will ultimately find gratitude for who you are and where you are."

He became very peaceful again.

Chapter 4

Survival Fears

Despite these new moments of peace, Vaughn admitted that he often wasn't happy, but didn't know what to do about it. He thought his difficulties were his fault and was blaming himself for his situation. He felt insecure, afraid of judgment, and overly concerned about how others saw him. He carried a sense of powerlessness and hopeless despair that his life was destined to be unfulfilling and miserable.

Despite that, he demonstrated enormous courage in coming to each session willing to learn, to become more self-aware, and to question every belief he thought was real. One day he showed up in an agitated state. His body was tense, his movements erratic, he was pale, nervous and jumpy. His anxiety levels were high and the sounds he was making expressed how disturbed he was. He typed that he was terrified that he wasn't safe because he couldn't speak and wasn't independent enough.

I thanked him for having the courage to show me through his energy, body language and typing how afraid he was. I assured

The Beautiful Language of the Heart

him that I didn't underestimate his daily challenges with non-speaking autism. Nor did I compare his journey to that of anyone else. After he was sure I understood the difficulties of his situation, I let him know that he was not the only one with survival fears.

"Everybody has their own version of intense survival fears, for their own reasons. It can be about a lack of emotional or physical safety, health, finances, love, self-worth, or death, to name a few. These fears can be accompanied by intense anxiety, depression, or powerlessness and can be quite debilitating."

Vaughn was relieved to know he wasn't the only one with survival fears. He was surprised that many of the deep issues he was facing actually had to do with being human and not specifically with autism. "It's a human thing, not only an autism thing" became a phrase I repeated to him quite often.

He became extremely interested in understanding what everyone faces on their journey, because he was already more than familiar with the specifics of his autism. I continued to flesh out the picture by letting him know that all of these fears, no matter what they are about, have some things in common.

These fears tell us there's danger that can harm us which we are powerless to handle. They say we are not good enough, don't have enough, and are never doing enough. They say we are solely responsible for making our life work. They demand that we exert more control over our lives. They say it's solely up to us to figure out what to do, and only then will our circumstances improve.

"Vaughn, the perspective of being in survival is extremely stressful and creates tension in your body, like you're feeling right now. At the root of all survival fears is fear that we don't have, or are separate from, what we most need. These needs include safety, support, abundance, love, respect, dignity, belonging, self-worth, power, possibilities, and connectedness.

"For a child, the concern is, 'Am I getting enough?' For an adolescent it's, 'Am I good enough?' For a young adult it's, 'Am I doing enough?'

For a healthy adult it's, 'Yes, I am connected, full and grateful.'

"For some people, survival fears can feel like being in an emergency situation with their inner alarm system blaring, always looking for what could go wrong. For others, they can feel terrified that their needs will never be met, or powerless because it seems like life will never work. Some people collapse in hopeless despair and give up on life. Others go into fight mode to hurry up and do something to get their needs met. They try harder and harder, trying to be more powerful, yet end up stressed and exhausted from the enormous pressure. Others freeze and feel paralyzed without options."

Vaughn nodded knowingly in recognition of the pressure, stress and anxiety he was feeling in his body.

Vaughn's father Ryan sat next to him with his hand lightly resting on his back during all of our sessions. Ryan valued participating in Vaughn's sessions because he got to know Vaughn's inner world better. At the start of each session, Ryan was eager to know what Vaughn would type. There were always fascinating surprises regarding what he wanted to discuss. Ryan's presence was also very reassuring to Vaughn, which helped him type more easily.

Since this session was about survival fears, I asked Ryan to touch the base of Vaughn's head in the back where our reptilian

The Beautiful Language of the Heart

brain, or amygdala, is located. This part of our brain is where survival fears come from, I told him. Survival perspectives are hardwired into our nervous system and it's easy for that primitive part of us to get triggered.

I explained to Vaughn that when we think we're in a survival situation, even when we're not, our body tenses, preparing for fight, flight or freeze. Then our body produces all of the necessary biochemistry as if we're preparing for war or famine, even when that's not actually what's happening.

Over time, this has an enormously wearing impact on our body, our emotions, and our mental and physical health. It's ultimately damaging to stay in a state of red alert as if we're always in a state of emergency. Even when we're not actually in a survival situation, we're so programmed to think we are, that we don't fully relax and feel safe. We're always waiting for something to go wrong or for "the other shoe to drop."

Vaughn nodded vigorously to let me know his survival fear was being understood. I asked him what scared him so much. He answered that he was afraid of getting lost and would never be able to get home because he doesn't speak. He feared that even if someone found him, due to being without speech, he wouldn't be able to identify himself by giving his name and address.

"Even though your fear seems so real, what if lack of safety is not the only possibility?" I invited Vaughn to reconsider the two beliefs that he couldn't communicate because he didn't have speech, and that he wasn't safe.

He was surprised and amazed when I let him know that he was already communicating excellently in nonverbal ways with his energy, body language, and also through typing. "Vaughn, your energy and emotions are so extraordinarily transparent and readily available that it's easier for me to communicate with you than with most people."

*I was inviting him
to change his perspective.*

"What if we can always choose a new perspective, which lets us deeply relax, and also allows for multiple positive solutions we might not have thought of? In your example of getting lost, what if your new perspective could include that you are safe and can communicate even without speech? Or what if your parents found you even though you couldn't give your name and address? Or what if you felt safe even if you were lost and as a result found your way home? Or what if you didn't get lost in the first place? What if you're actually safe? How would you feel?"

He lit up and relaxed when he started to realize that he was already communicating and safe. His body softened, color and light came in his face and eyes, and a big smile crossed his face. "Ah, there you are! I can see you now beyond your survival fear. Bravo Vaughn!"

Vaughn was very interested in finding out how this kind of change in his feeling state happened.

"In this session you had an experience of changing your point of view. You shifted from the anxiety of imagined danger in the future, to feeling safe right here, right now, in the present, sitting in your chair. You relaxed into an inner resonance field of safety when you realized that you're actually safe. Can you see how that change in perspective changed your whole outlook and feeling state?"

"I feel so much lighter and freer. There's hope now."

"Which do you like better, the anxiety or the lightness?" I winked at him.

"Inner lightness and freedom create a much safer outer life in general. Then, if there ever was some danger to respond to, you would be able to much more effectively from this relaxed open place, rather than from paralyzing panic."

Since he had experienced the change in his feelings and outlook right away, he wanted to be able to do that himself next time he felt anxious. He asked me to teach him how to do that. "You're so good at this stuff," he typed. I had a belly laugh over the way "this stuff" nicely summarized my life's work about the nature of reality, existence, and human consciousness.

"Many people are motivated to heal because they're suffering or in crisis. When we are in pain and without hope, it seems like if we could just change our outer life circumstances, we'd feel better. It seems that it's only our circumstances that are causing our pain. In your case, it seems like if you could change the autism or could just speak, you'd feel safe and happy. There are some circumstances we can change and some we can't, but in either case, you can always change your point of view."

Vaughn wanted to know what a new point of view might be.

"We can change our perspective from hopelessness to hope, for example. Then, despite extraordinarily challenging situations with no obvious solutions, we are valiant spirits who can meet those challenges when we have hope. Hope uplifts us to a new point of view that reveals possibilities and solutions that may not have been visible before. Having hope and possibility instead of hopeless impossibility represents a change in perspective."

Vaughn stared off into the distance for a long time, contemplating what I was saying. A slight smile crossed his face as he was considering hope.

"When we feel powerless and despairing, it seems that there's no other possibility. But just because you feel powerless, it doesn't mean you are powerless. Just because you feel hopeless, it doesn't mean there isn't hope.

"Most people think that change is only about altering our external reality. However, our perspective is really what changes first. When we change our perspective, our inner feelings change, we see reality differently, and then we can make the necessary changes to bring our outer life into harmony with our new point of view."

Vaughn was interested in knowing how this works.

"When our perceptions and perspectives change, so does our consciousness along with its energy, frequencies, beliefs, thoughts, emotions, and sensations. As our consciousness itself deepens and expands, we experience a new resonance field, which is a new state of being.

"For a new perspective to become real in our lives, it must be more than just a good idea. It's not just an intellectual change in perspective that's needed. For a new perspective to become authentically embodied, we need to feel the relief, lightness, and freedom of it in our body.

"When we feel this lightness deeply enough, it becomes real for us. Its frequencies uplift us to a higher level of consciousness. This not only changes the way we feel, but also empowers us to make positive changes in our lives. It's like breaking a bad habit and living from a healthier place, which gradually becomes the new reality.

Vaughn started to see what a profound change it would be for him to live from relaxed safety rather than the chronic anxiety of believing he's always at risk. He hadn't known that his underlying state of being had been anxiety producing inherent danger instead of relaxing inherent safety.

In addition to perception of constant danger, lack of love is another fear-based story that Vaughn often faced. Even though he's a very open person when it comes to being loving, he couldn't take in how deeply loved he is. I told him again and again how much I appreciate and cherish him, but at first he wouldn't take it in. My words bounced off of his defenses because he didn't believe he was worthy of love.

Even though he had been negatively judged persistently, he realized that he was continuing to perpetuate and perpetrate that cruelty on himself. As he came face to face with his own self-rejecting belief that he wasn't good enough, he could feel how harsh and unkind that was. He discovered that what he really wanted was to be kind to himself.

After this realization, he was more able to receive my appreciation and began to express his gratitude in return. His expressions of thanks were so palpable and sincere, they pierced my heart. When I let him know the powerful impact of his love, I was inviting him to keep changing his perspective from flat to round.

Vaughn also typed that he felt an extreme amount of pressure that was depressing. He thought it was up to him to handle, control and manage everything. Because he believed he was solely responsible for making his life work, he carried the weight of the world on his shoulders. He became overwhelmed and despairing, because he couldn't do what he thought he should. He was trying to control everything in order to be perfect, powerful and never vulnerable, which he didn't realize would be impossible for anyone.

"Vaughn, the illusion of separation is the fundamental misperception of flat consciousness and gives rise to our fear-based stories. When we think we're separate, we try to be in charge of All That Is and control life. But since we're part of, and connected with All That Is, the concept of being in charge of it doesn't actually make any sense. Within the perspective of separation, it seems like 'I'm over here, my higher self is over there, my soul and spirit are elsewhere and 'God' is far outside of me.' Then we supposedly get together at a big table and negotiate.

"What if you're already connected, safe, and supported and just have been living with the misperception that you're alone and it's all up to you?"

He heaved a big sigh of relief as he typed, "All of the pressure just came off. I feel so different!"

"The possibility that there can be new perspectives which we can choose and explore is a new perspective in itself. Choice itself is empowering. Change is about choice and hope. When we free ourselves up enough to understand that we do have choice, we get to explore what we really want to choose."

We always have the freedom
to choose
a new perspective.

Chapter 5
Feeling All Feelings

Vaughn often started our conversations by typing about things that he couldn't do, the outbursts he would have, and why he was angry and frustrated with himself. As he typed his emotions, he would express them with specific sounds and gestures. Gradually, I got to know what each one meant.

One day, after expressing a lot of understandable anger and frustration, he jumped up and ran out of the room. He was withdrawing in shame for having shown intense emotion. Like so many people, Vaughn had been taught to suppress his feelings rather than feeling them, and letting their energy flow.

He was embarrassed that he had such strong reactions to trivial situations. He typed that he hated forks. When he saw one, he would grab it off the table and replace it with chopsticks. He looked down at the floor with a red flush of shame on his face.

"Vaughn, I understand the intensity of your feelings, which most likely originated in past trauma and did not start with forks. For instance, do you think a fork can hurt someone's mouth?

Does the thought of a wounded mouth remind you of the time when you were little, fell down, split your lip badly, and got rushed to the hospital to get stitches?"

"Yes!" He was excited about understanding this. "I'm afraid that a fork will poke a hole in my mom's cheek. I would never want her to go through what I did when I fell and split my lip. There was a lot of blood and trauma, and when I was in the hospital, I thought I was going to another place, as in dying. It was terrifying."

"When feelings are very intense and get triggered by a seemingly trivial thing like forks, they can stem from an early trauma like you had. Or they can build over time so you end up feeling like you're in a pressure cooker. You haven't known it's ok to express your anger as it comes up, so you're probably scared that the pressure cooker is going to explode?"

He nodded with the relief of being understood.

"I know how caring your heart is. You would never want to hurt anyone if your anger exploded, so it got turned inward into depression. The same happened with your fear, which turned inward into anxiety. So, no matter how trivial the current situation, it's important to express, not suppress, your feelings. They're pointing to something in you that is calling for healing."

As Vaughn started becoming more trusting that his feelings were being accepted, he became less frightened of them. He was able to express his emotions without running out of the room. When they got intense, he would still jump up out of his chair at times, but was able to sit right back down and stay with what he was feeling. Ryan's guiding touch on Vaughn's arm or back was extremely helpful in reassuring him that he was ok.

The Beautiful Language of the Heart

"Vaughn, almost everybody has been taught that it's not acceptable to have certain feelings or to express the full range of them. Everybody has wanted to run away from their feelings at some point in life. But, all feelings are valuable because if we turn off one feeling, then we turn off the broad range of our feelings, which includes happiness and joy. Living within a limited range of feelings is like being an artist who can paint with only one color, or a musician who can play only one note."

He nodded vigorously, letting me know he understood.

Since Vaughn was very gifted at feeling subtle energies, we started talking about feelings as energy in his body. He noticed that when he expressed his emotions, their energy moved through his body effortlessly and he relaxed immediately. He discovered that feeling his feelings is empowering, whereas rejecting and judging them shut him down and turned off the flow of energy.

Vaughn began to see how he habitually shut down his feelings. He noticed that he would push away and retreat into repetitive mental loops in his head that were some kind of fear-based stories about the future. One of his most painful stories was, "I'll never have a girlfriend because I'm broken. No one will ever want to be close to me." Since he believed his story was real, he became terrified that he would be alone forever.

"Instead of being so sure that your future is bleak, which shuts you down, what about opening up to connect from your heart? That lets your inner light shine, which is totally gorgeous and attractive."

I invited him to play a little game with me, which piqued his curiosity. I asked him to feel the difference between shutting down and opening up. "When you shut down, have you noticed that you contract, get tense, wall off, and feel pressure in your body? Do you notice that you withdraw and hide deep inside, put up walls of defense, or leave your body?"

"Yes, all of those, and they feel terrible."

"Shutting down causes pain in the body," I suggested.

"My stomach is clenched in a tight knot right now. It hurts."

"What happens in your body when you let your feelings move?" I asked.

"I'm starting to see that feeling feelings is not terrifying. When I'm thinking about a feeling instead of actually feeling the energy of it, it persists. Then I don't have a sense of relief. When I actually feel the feeling, there's an expansion and the tension resolves." He took a deep breath and felt his stomach relax.

I explained to him that authentic feelings have a palpable sensation of flow, vibration and light-filled aliveness. They resonate. Authentic feeling is natural and feels good because it's pure energy in motion, with no beliefs or stories attached. Authentic feelings are soft and move easily, rich with their own unique vibration, which is palpable. When we allow them to move through us as pure energy, they empower us.

When we feel our feelings
and let the energy move,
we change

When we restrict, reject, or judge ourselves we block the flow, like a logjam in the river. Eventually, more and more energy concentrates around the logjam, which further reduces our natural flow. This cuts off our power and is why we feel stuck.

The Beautiful Language of the Heart

Vaughn began to ask for my help in letting his feelings flow when he found that he was shut down. When he came into a session with severe anxiety, I would remind him to slow down, breathe, move out of his mental stories, and come back into his heart. There, he found peace and calm once again.

A few minutes later, he jumped up and made anxious sounds. Ryan reached for Vaughn's hand to comfort him, and he sat back down. Vaughn wanted to know why the peace went away. I assured him that even though it feels like it leaves, it never goes away. We are the ones who forget it's there and move away from it. We go somewhere else, usually into our head. As we remember to come back down into our body, be present and open up, we experience its flow again.

As Vaughn got more comfortable with expressing his feelings, he realized that every emotion, sensation and feeling is valuable. We are taught that some emotions are good and some are bad, while some are right and some are wrong. In either case, we're taught not to express them too fully if at all. We are taught to control our emotions instead of feeling them flow and letting them empower us.

Emotion is a continuous flow that is constantly shifting and changing. There's no hierarchy of better or worse emotions. All are of equal importance, and all are an integral part of our wholeness.

We are

an

ocean

of

Anamika

sensations
feelings
emotions
and
thoughts
constantly moving
and
changing.

As we welcome the full range of our emotions and feelings, they expand our inner fullness, which is limitless and goes on forever.

Feeling the full range of our feelings
does not incapacitate us.
It empowers us
impacts All That Is
and
together
we become more.

Chapter 6

Experiencing Ourselves

One day I asked Vaughn who he is. "I am a man who wants to live my life from beauty and grace." He was yearning to experience himself beyond the pain and suffering that were coming from recycling mental loops and false beliefs about himself.

I explained to him that who we truly are is so much more expansive than we've ever known or can ever understand. We are far greater than our "ordinary" self. Who we are extends far beyond our body and our personality. Our true nature is multidimensional and limitless, which is so vast that it also includes our limited three-dimensional self.

We've tried to know ourselves by answering the age-old question, "Who am I?" We can describe our appearance, likes and dislikes, personality traits, skills and talents, as well as what we do. But, we cannot describe who we are. It's not something we can define intellectually.

When we focus only on our limitations and what we can't do,

we suffer. By contrast, our limitless nature is expansive, active, dynamic and ever-changing. It's full of hope, possibility and joy.

The uncharted territory of our limitless nature is something the rational mind alone can never comprehend, but it can be deeply felt and experienced. While the linear mind wants to understand, explain and define, our larger self says, "Go experience, because intellectual understanding alone isn't adequate to describe the poetry of the heart."

Since we can't know ourselves only with our mind, and since the experience of our limitlessness doesn't have language, how can we know ourselves?

*A new kind of language is needed,
the beautiful language of the heart.*

Being with Vaughn was always joyous for me because one of the gifts of his autism is that he doesn't have thick filters to get through to reach him. He's extraordinarily open, transparent, and able to feel not only his own energy, but everyone else's too. That made it easy to guide him out of his mental loops and into his felt experience.

We can become aware of experiencing ourselves during unexpected moments of expansion in which we feel exquisite love, beauty, or freedom. When a baby smiles, emotions well up in us and our heart expands with love. Music moves us and our body reverberates with resonance. It's palpable. It flows.

In those moments, we are experiencing the aspect of us that is always there underneath everything else. For a brief moment, we touch it. We resonate with what's deeply within and around

The Beautiful Language of the Heart

us, and we enter its flow. Suddenly, we're seeing through different eyes that are softer and more clear. We feel alive and free.

We tingle with
waves
of
warmth
substance
movement
light.

We open into the part of us that our physical eyes can't see and our ears can't hear. Yet, we sense and recognize it as our real self. It's undefinable, but we can experience it beyond our common senses. Through our uncommon senses, we are able to perceive the energy that vibrates and resonates beyond the ordinary.

When we identify only with our body or personality, we experience ourselves as finite. The finite world can be measured and quantified. But when we feel the movement of our energy, substance, warmth, and light forever expanding, we are identifying with our infinite nature, which includes the finite.

It's thrilling as we're expanding into the lightness and freedom beyond what we already know. Yet, we can also feel threatened and scared at the same time. That's understandable because the limited finite self thinks that it's the one who defines who we are. It holds on tightly to its finite sense of self because it can't perceive what's infinite. Moreover, what's infinite can't be captured, contained or explained. It can only be experienced as we explore its vastness.

Anamika

When experiencing,
the air thickens
our thoughts slow down
and
we become aware of the space
between our thoughts.
We taste and touch
something beyond our ordinary self.
As we enter the mystery
we experience
unspeakable intimacy
with
all of existence.
This moving, pulsating aliveness
is who we are.
We are extraordinarily and magnificently
complex
yet simple and natural
when experienced.

Our consciousness is aware of itself, and grows in that awareness the more we're present with it. Through our ability to see and feel ourselves with clarity, we are constantly transcending ourselves and becoming more.

Our consciousness can't be
contained
explained
captured

The Beautiful Language of the Heart

or put in a box.
It can only be experienced
for the joy of it.

Chapter 7

Starting to Accept Himself

Vaughn was self-conscious about his autism and had a long history of frustrating experiences as a child. When I first asked him what life was like when he was young, he got agitated and ran out of the room. When he finally came back of his own accord, Beth wisely let him know that everyone has trouble facing some of their childhood feelings. Ryan praised him for his courage and willingness to discuss his past.

I asked Vaughn what the most difficult part of his childhood had been. He said he was always feeling bad about himself because he couldn't easily do things teachers asked him to, like stacking cups. He felt like an utterly incapable failure.

I suggested that everyone learns in different ways and he needed to be approached in a way that might have worked better for him. He was expected to fit into a set program that wasn't attuned to his personal learning style. The program demanded things of him that he couldn't do. So, despite his sharp intellect

The Beautiful Language of the Heart

and creative gifts, learning for Vaughn became an enraging chore instead of an enjoyable discovery.

We went back in time to some of those scenes. I asked him to imagine being approached by teachers in a way that honored his rare sensitivities and gifts. First, he lit up with joy as he imagined being accepted. Then a wave of sadness crossed his face when he realized how much better his life would have been. My heart ached as I felt what he had been through. "I'm so sorry about your past experiences, but it's not too late to learn to feel good about yourself now."

Vaughn had a lifetime of being subjected to extreme judgment from other people, who looked at him as if there was something wrong with him. After gently acknowledging the severity of what he had experienced, it helped when I let him know that these issues were not unique to him. They are human issues people face at different levels of intensity, for different reasons, and in their own way. It was reassuring to him when I let him know that everyone has been judged and has a fear of judgment. "It's a human thing not just an autism thing."

To give him a taste of what was possible beyond judgment, I told him how I saw him. "You are smart, capable and strong enough to be vulnerable. You are extraordinary. No matter how bad it's been, you never gave up. You always found forgiveness and sought more love. You're courageous and humble enough to keep growing. I honor your dignity and character. You're already the kind of man you told me you want to be, 'a man of beauty and grace.'"

He couldn't believe that he was already full of beauty and grace. He was stunned that he could be accepted exactly as he was, especially because of the limitations of his autism. "Vaughn, your particular path is no accident and your life is not a mistake, nor are you. There's nothing wrong with anything about you, including your autism. In time, you're going to see the gifts of your autism as well as the beauty of your path."

Vaughn's eyes grew wide in amazement. "Your autism provides you with both gifts and limitations. That's also a human thing, not just an autism thing. We each have our gifts and limitations, and although you have autism, it is not who you are. You are you, you are beautiful you."

Vaughn shook his head from side to side vigorously as if he couldn't believe what he was hearing. Then he lit up with elation as he realized that he was a beautiful being; he was not his autism. The autism was something he had, but it isn't who he is as a person.

Gradually, he could see that autism had developed some extraordinary capacities in him. It took appreciating the very thing he thought was wrong with him to begin to feel himself underneath the autism. Week after week, I helped him touch his real self as we became still, breathed together, and he dropped into his body. In the inner silence, he could feel his real self beyond his personality and deeper than the autism. In the stillness, he could feel that he was uniquely and perfectly Vaughn.

Every time his face took on an especially transcendent look, Ryan and I would immediately feel Vaughn's energy shift, and would shoot each other a delighted glance through the Zoom screen. It was lovely sharing our mutual appreciation as Vaughn exuded his glorious light, filling the room.

Vaughn's sensitivity to sensing energy and his capacity to

The Beautiful Language of the Heart

radiate it are exceptional. Due to this gift of sensitivity, he realized that his inner young boy and his present day grown-up self both needed to be approached with great awareness and care.

During the exercise with the imaginary teachers, he got to heal his inner young boy by imagining being approached with tenderness. This led into a conversation about the fact that we are all made of many parts. We are not just one "I" like a bottle of homogenized milk. I asked him to picture a bottle of white milk and then picture a beef stew with chunks of meat, carrots and potatoes floating in a broth. We are like the stew with many parts within us: a child, an adolescent, a young adult, an adult, a positive ego, a negative ego with its mental loops, a finite self, an infinite self, and so much more. Each has its own point of view, which is sometimes in conflict with the others, and sometimes in harmony.

We can access all of our inner parts and get to know their feelings, wounds, and needs. We can heal what never got healed. Like instruments in an orchestra, each part of us keeps its own unique identity while interrelating with the greater whole. As each part heals, it comes into harmony with the whole orchestra to create a magnificent symphony.

There's nothing bad about any of our parts or their feelings. When we receive their pain with love and compassion, they get integrated and outgrow acting out their unhealed pain. We can't get rid of any parts of ourselves, as much as we might want to. But they can be understood, healed, and integrated.

We're not broken
and
we don't need to be fixed.

Anamika

The more we try to fix and perfect ourselves, the more we suffer. It hurts when we blame, shame, or exile any part of ourselves. When we hold each part in tender love and acceptance without pressuring it to change, it feels valued as part of the whole.

Every part of us is valuable
acceptable
and precious for what it is.
It longs to be illuminated
not eliminated.

Appreciating all of our parts for what they contribute is part of integrating and enlightening. In that interdependent relationship, we come into greater harmony.

Every part of us
yearns to bask
in the light
of our tender regard.
Our heart is vast enough
to hold All.
We thrive in
our love's
compassionate
embrace.

As Vaughn began to accept himself more, he began to feel happier. At one point he got confused and thought he had to hold onto the happiness so he could feel that way all the time.

The Beautiful Language of the Heart

I let him know that he didn't need to be happy or positive all of the time. It doesn't work to push away from what we're actually feeling at any given moment by trying to be happy. Just be in this present moment, I advised.

Happiness comes from self-acceptance.
The more present and accepting we are,
the happier we become.

As Vaughn was beginning to accept himself, he was breaking through his chronic isolation. He began to feel hopeful that his life could change.

Chapter 8

Feeling Connected

Every night before saying goodnight to Vaughn, Ryan repeated a little ritual. He named Vaughn's lovely qualities, and each time he got to the word "connected," Vaughn lit up. His exuberant response to that word made it clear that feeling connected was one of the feelings he yearned for the most.

In his great desire to connect, Vaughn would grab Ryan around the back of the neck. Being a big strong guy, sometimes his grip was vigorous. It looked uncomfortable for Ryan, so I asked Vaughn why he was grabbing his dad's neck. He said it was to feel closer to his father.

I explained to him that feeling close comes from the heart, not from the neck. I invited him to send a beam of light from his heart to his father's heart. I invited Ryan to do the same in return. Within a very short time, the two of them were in bliss, feeling closer to each other than ever before.

Ryan commented that he could really feel Vaughn on a whole new level. That new level was the depth of connection Vaughn

The Beautiful Language of the Heart

had been seeking. Vaughn looked very content and fulfilled and stopped grabbing Ryan's neck, at least for the moment.

Despite craving closeness, making eye contact was hard for Vaughn. One day I noticed him peek at me on the Zoom screen. I let him know how wonderful that felt to me. I was curious to know how it felt to him. He typed, "I'm graciously enraptured." His words shot an arrow of love directly into my heart. His unique way of expressing himself never failed to touch me.

I asked him how he feels in his body when he takes a peek and we feel each other's energy. "Content and deeply connected and finally fulfilled." His face lit up with the joy of feeling a depth of relating that reached his heart and soul. I addressed him with the utmost tenderness, "Hi, Vaughn." I paused and repeated, "Hi, Vaughn. What happens when I say hi to you?" He felt our connection immediately and responded, "Overwhelmed with happiness and joy and gratitude."

I gently persisted, "Where do you go inside yourself to feel that?" He answered without thought or hesitation as if it was the most natural thing in the world, "I just focus on my heart, and that's it. I'm getting better at that now."

When we think of connecting, perhaps we imagine a bond with other people, animals or nature. These are certainly invaluable. But it goes much deeper than that. Connecting is not only about with whom we are connecting but from what part of us. Is it superficial? Is it deep? Is it from our inner child, our adolescent? Our heart and soul? Our entire being?

When we come from the heart and surrender our sense of separateness, we feel warm, close, and a part of instead of apart from. But that feeling of connection doesn't require anyone to make it happen for us. It's an internal experience, a flow of energy, a state of being.

Have you ever been with people and felt even more alone? That's because the inner energy flow wasn't flowing. Or, have you ever been in solitude and felt whole, complete and fulfilled? That happens when the inner flow of energy is flowing and we're in a state of being of connectedness.

In this flow of energy
we feel deeply connected to ourselves
to everyone and everything everywhere
and to All That Is.
Each precious moment
of connecting
changes us forever.

Our desire to experience more and more connection is not just the longing of our heart, but of our entire being. We long to know more of who we are and of All That Is. The heart doesn't control or force, it feels. It calls, beckons and patiently invites. Our yearning heeds that call, gently guiding us beyond separation and disconnection.

"When I was very young, I felt connected to my parents, and then it went away. Then, you helped me get reconnected and now I'm afraid it's going to go away again. I've been having recurring nightmares of being all alone," Vaughn disclosed.

"The good news is that you're already completely connected and can never actually be disconnected, even though at times you might feel alone. It's easy to forget that we are all interconnected

The Beautiful Language of the Heart

in a field of love that we are one with, so we can never actually be alone," I assured him.

"By saying that, you have helped me with these nightmares." He heaved a sigh of relief.

"Also, Vaughn, feeling alone and disconnected is a human thing, not only an autism thing," I reminded him. Ryan nodded that he sometimes feels that way too. "That's good to hear because I can forget quickly and think it's my autism."

"When you remember that you're eternally connected, where do you feel that in your body?" I asked.

"In my entire body. When I'm in that state, my chest and head are relaxed and calm," he replied peacefully, "and I trust that my needs are met, so I don't panic."

Through our heart
our whole body
and our whole being
we feel vastly expansive
interrelated
and connected
to everything everywhere.
The more we connect
the more peaceful and content
we become
and
the more alive we feel.

"When you're feeling connected, Vaughn, I'll bet you don't long for it anymore, because it's already there. The more you

Anamika

trust that it's always there, it becomes more intensely intimate and seems more real. It's an eternal process, not a goal that you finally achieve."

*Connectedness
is our natural state.
It's always there
within everything.
We don't suddenly find it.
It's been in us
all along.
We can sense its warmth
by slipping into the ineffable mystery
and indefinable depths
where words
ideas
thoughts
and definitions
cannot go.
We touch
the richness
and the
beautiful expansive complexity
through which we
and all that exists
become more.
Connecting is a continual luminous expansion
in unimaginable directions simultaneously
like a star going supernova.*

The Beautiful Language of the Heart

You experience yourself
as consciousness
getting to know itself more.
Connecting is a veritable romance
with ourselves, others, and All.

As we begin connecting at more expansive levels, we start to experience our multidimensional nature. We get to know ourselves both as our own unique consciousness and as also as connected to the greater whole.

In embracing our limited nature
as well as our limitlessness
we evolve.

When connecting, we don't lose our individual self. To the contrary, the more connected to the infinite, the more we experience who we are individually. Then, the more we experience who we are individually, the more connected we feel.

Even though we are seemingly just one person who is separate from everything else, quantum physics has revealed our interconnectedness. This means that we are simultaneously our individual selves and also interconnected with all. It's the paradox of and/and.

Most people identify only as finite beings who occasionally touch the infinite. Flat. In the new paradigm of consciousness, we identify as infinite beings who express in the finite for the joy of it. Round.

The infinite is more than big enough to hold the finite. In its

Anamika

limitless expansiveness, we feel at one with ourselves and simultaneously with all that exists.

All is so much more
than we now know
or will ever know.
All is always becoming more
and more means
it has never existed before.

We are always growing
evolving
and expanding.
So is All That Is.
We can relish the richness
of what is right now
even while desiring more.

We are a mystery
longing to be further explored.
We are a fluid, dynamic process
continually becoming.
We are an unlimited, continuous flow
of unfolding and enfolding complexity
beyond rational comprehension
but not beyond experience.

We are consciousness
exploring and discovering itself

The Beautiful Language of the Heart

*becoming more
reverberating with resonance
creating and expanding
infinitely.
Our consciousness is connected to
everyone everything everywhere
as one
in love with
everyone everything everywhere.*

Chapter 9

Gentle and Forgiving

Vaughn had spent many years feeling disappointed in himself for not being more capable and independent. He had put a lot of pressure on himself to be more "advanced" than he was at any given moment. As a result, he was constantly mad at himself.

I suggested gentleness and forgiveness toward himself rather than punishing pressure. I explained to him that self-forgiveness doesn't mean he has done anything wrong or isn't far enough along. "You don't have to believe you've done something wrong or you're not far enough along in order to benefit from self-forgiveness and kindness towards yourself. It's more like an acknowledgment that although you've been hard on yourself, you care enough about yourself to be more gentle from here on."

He liked the idea and gradually began to shift from the harshness of self-judgment to the gentleness of self-forgiveness. While this felt wonderful to him, he was worried because after blissful moments of peace, the anxiety and frustration would return. I

The Beautiful Language of the Heart

explained to him that change is not a linear process.

We go back and forth and back and forth, which can feel quite topsy-turvy. The process can be messy as we alternate between opening and closing, expanding and contracting, relaxing and tensing, remembering and forgetting, or clarity and confusion. We go back and forth between resonance and dissonance, feeling in sync and out of sync.

I asked him to imagine an orchestra warming up. "Can you hear the screeches of the violin and the booming of the bass? That cacophony is dissonance. After they warm up, they come into harmony to play a gorgeous symphony. Harmony is a new resonance that comes after the dissonance."

I asked him to imagine an upward spiral:

Dissonance → Resonance

Resonance → Dissonance

Dissonance → Greater resonance

Greater resonance → Further dissonance

→ Even greater resonance

"Vaughn, we tend to think of one as good and the other as bad. But, peace comes from embracing both of these polarities. It's and/and, not either/or. They are both part of the process. This means that there's nothing wrong with where you are."

Vaughn liked when I reminded him about being patient, gentle and forgiving with himself for who you are and where you are. I sang him a silly little Double Yammy song, " I yam who I yam, I yam where I yam." As soon as I mentioned these things, he relaxed, took the unnecessary pressure off himself, and sank into a gentler place. He felt better immediately and stopped struggling with himself to be ahead of where he was.

He began to realize that he was shaming, blaming and driving himself to be "perfect." Perfectionism and self-punishment were causing his anxiety. "When we're relaxed and at peace we grow and progress naturally, without pushing or forcing. Have you ever seen an athlete in the zone? They're relaxed while performing the most incredible feats!"

He often asked me to remind him of "progress not perfection," the need for repetition, and gentle forgivingness regarding bumps along the way." He felt better knowing that nobody's path was smooth, and that growth is a lifelong process. It never ends and we are never finished learning, exploring, and discovering.

Vaughn also enjoyed having me challenge his negative beliefs by asking if he'd be willing to be "wrong" about his point of view. I clarified that wrong doesn't mean bad, it means limited. At first, he resisted because he was so sure he was right about how unlovable he was. Eventually, he enjoyed reconsidering his fear-based perspectives, and discovered the joy and wonder of being "wrong."

After he felt safe with his beliefs being wrong, he admitted that he was bored with his mental loops and their repetitive negative beliefs. Staying in those loops was not a fun place to be, he concluded.

To me, his boredom indicated he was ready to explore more of the unknown. "It definitely gets boring if we only stay with what we already know. Many people can stretch beyond what we know to what we know that we don't know. But the thrill of

The Beautiful Language of the Heart

life is when we open to what we don't know that we don't know. This requires being willing to enter the unknown."

We talked about the linear mind wanting to know everything ahead of time, thinking that's how we stay safe. Flat. Then there's the adventure of exploration and discovery within the unknown. Round.

We can't control what's unknown, but we can relate to it with curiosity, openness, and appreciation. Through discovery, what was unknown becomes known, and there's always more unknown to discover.

All That Is
yearns to engage with us
just as we yearn
to experience All.

When we're willing to enter the unknown, we can't force ourselves to let go of what we currently know. But we can gently slip below the surface of what we've known. Despite any fears, we won't drown or lose ourselves. We will actually find more.

I invited him to contemplate some new perspectives:

I'm willing to find out who I am
beyond who I currently think I am.
I'm willing to look beyond what I think I want or need.
I'm willing to consider that reality
is more than I can
currently or ever
imagine.
I'm willing to be open

Anamika

to ongoing discovery.

*Discovery
is
our soul's call
to adventure.*

Vaughn loved the idea of exploring and discovering but admitted that he got scared and angry when his daily routines changed. He knew that this was a contradiction and was sure that fear of change was due to his autism.

"I really hear you when you say that autism makes this more extreme for you. For some people it can definitely be much harder than for others. But at some level change can be hard for everyone. So, remember our favorite phrase: It's a human thing, not just an autism thing.

"The reason it's challenging for everyone is because embracing change is about giving up control. We're taught we must take control to make life work. But, change and control can't exist at the same time because control is an attempt to keep things the same, or within what's already known, rather than breaking free."

To experiment with giving up control, we tried a little exercise. "Imagine your third-dimensional limited self saying, 'It's out of my hands. My life is none of my business. Since opportunity is my natural state of being, I don't have to try hard to make life happen. I can receive effortlessly from my infinite self and All That Is.'"

Vaughn laughed with relief at no longer having to control everything. He wanted to freely explore, while also being aware of his fears, since fear and dread tend to accompany change.

The Beautiful Language of the Heart

He felt relieved when he was free from being imprisoned by trying to control and fix his life. He felt elated by the resulting lightness and freedom.

There is freedom
from
and freedom
into.
Freedom from restriction
is a good start.
But the more profound change occurs
with freedom into lightness.

Freedom *from* our negativity lifts us out of what we don't want. Instead of staying stuck in what we've believed, we're now available to engage freedom *into*. It's a lighter, more expansive feeling that opens into infinite possibility.

Freedom happens when we stretch beyond thinking any particular idea is the *only* truth. When we can include more than our version of what's "right" and "real," we find the joy, wonder, and surprise inherent in freedom.

Freedom is an unbridled feeling
of
floating in weightlessness
where
you can't fall
because
there's no gravity anymore.

Chapter 10

Self-Love

Vaughn showed up to his next session happy and peaceful. I asked him what had changed. "My disability doesn't define me anymore." This was a huge breakthrough for him.

"I'm having a change of focus and I'm thinking differently about myself. I can be recognized for myself now and not limited by my autism."

He acknowledged that some days were harder than others in remembering this new perspective. "Sometimes I forget where I put it." I laughed at his humorous way of expressing profound things. I reassured him that sometimes I forget where I put it too. Ryan concurred and we all had a good laugh.

I reminded Vaughn again that being patient, gentle and loving toward himself was more important than getting to some imagined destination at warp speed.

"Slow down and remember to look for progress, not perfection, along with a good dose of self-acceptance and humor. It's wonderful when we can laugh at ourselves and not take life so seriously," I reminded him.

"These days it's getting easier to find joy by going to my heart," he responded.

As he was building more trust and comfort with the process, he began to talk about wanting to have a girlfriend. He was sure that could never happen. "Why not?" I countered.

I asked him how he would feel if he already had a girlfriend. "Loved and profoundly loving," he answered immediately.

"Why wait to feel that? Can you imagine feeling genuinely loved and profoundly loving right now? How would you feel if there's no lack of the love that you want?" The tension in his body released and the clench in his gut softened. His habitually anxious mind became still.

"What if the love you're seeking is already there inside of your heart?" I asked. "Rapture," was his immediate reply.

I invited him to consider that instead of waiting to have a girlfriend to feel loved, loving, and safe, he could go to that feeling right now. "When you go to your heart, which is always full of love, you feel wonderful. That naturally attracts people to you." With that reminder, he went right to his heart, which lit up and glowed. He was beaming with delight, overcome by the love he found there.

I asked Vaughn to choose an option: 1. Stay shut down in the certainty that your needs will never be met, or 2. Glow, receive and attract. His grin let me know that it was an obvious choice.

I told him that most people think that love comes from outside of themselves from someone else. They try hard to become worthy of earning that love by being successful enough, attractive enough, or perfect enough. They may go to drastic lengths to try to earn the love but may not end up feeling loved at all. Or, they are so afraid of losing love, they shut down and no longer feel it.

We tend to shut down when we get hurt. If a hurt is deep enough or sustained over time, we might want to stay shut down. It seems that keeping our heart shut down will keep us safe and protected from further hurt. While it can take time to heal traumas from the past, we can allow the present and future to be different than the past. We can consider learning to love and trust again.

Closing our hearts can also be based on the view that love is in short supply, it's hard to come by, and it only comes from another person. Flat.

When we focus on love coming from within, from an endless source, then it's always there and we can never lose it. In being present in our heart, we automatically feel loved and loving because that's our natural state of being. Round.

From that perspective, we can be open-hearted, open-minded, and undefended because we are inherently safe, lovable, and loved. When we let ourselves really feel that love and safety, it radiates out and positively impacts our life as well as the world.

"Vaughn, you are able to heal your hurts from the past. You're able to name them, feel the pain, and then choose to be open in the present. You can go to that beautiful heart of yours any time and feel its luscious energy radiating out connecting with everything and everyone everywhere.

"When you experience the love that's already there within you and all around, you don't need to wait to have a girlfriend to be 'in love.' You can go to your heart any time you want and share it, which is easy for you to do. Remember how many people are moved to tears when you hug them because they feel your radiant

The Beautiful Language of the Heart

love?" I was reminding Vaughn of stories Ryan had told me of the countless times grown men had melted in Vaughn's arms.

When we feel empty and in need of love, sometimes it can help to have someone's arms around us. But we can't actually fill that "hole" with their love. While someone else's love can help us relax, open, and remember that we're not alone, we're not dependent on that. When we open, whether with or without someone else's help, we immediately feel more of the fullness of our own heart shining.

A child is dependent on the love of others, so our inner child and adolescent will look to others for love. But as an adult, we can access our inner love in a way that we couldn't do as a child. As an adult, when we believe that we're still dependent on someone else giving us love, we're really saying that we are not whole in ourselves with more than enough love available. Inherently, we are already whole, so when we go within, we can feel the truth of our radiance.

"Vaughn, by letting your own love flow, you'll feel full and met. The more you focus on that and feel it, the more its intensity increases. It fulfills you and touches others. I am always moved by your love."

*Within and around us
is a wellspring of limitless love
from which we continually give and receive.
We are one with this wellspring.
True intimacy is when we're in this love
and simultaneously experiencing ourselves
as one with
this love.*

"Remember the four F's: Feeling first form follows. That means feel your own inner love first and then relationships will follow."

Vaughn's epiphany after this conversation was that his real desire was not to try to get love from someone else, but to feel his love radiating so he could share it with others. The more he expressed his own love, the closer he felt to others, and the more self-love he felt as well.

"I'm becoming my new best friend because I got tired of blaming myself for my disability. I'm not being down on myself now and I'm lighter of heart," Vaughn revealed.

"What does that feel like in your body?" I inquired. Ryan and I shot each other a delighted look because in answer to my question Vaughn was sitting there glowing like a megawatt light bulb.

"I'm really starting to feel good about myself!" he proclaimed.

Chapter 11
Understanding Life

*There is such
beauty and fragility
joy and sorrow
in being
human.*

After beginning to feel better about himself, Vaughn was eager to understand how life works. "What we've been taught about life and reality is the opposite of how it actually works. This is impossible for the mind to comprehend.

"Vaughn, let's take an example. You were conditioned to believe that you need to prove your worth. But what if that's not true? What if you already matter more than you can ever comprehend just because you exist as you?"

*Who we are is not
what we do.*

Anamika

*What we do
does not define
who we are.*

He looked at me, trying to comprehend how he could already matter. I guided him into his body to connect with the place inside in which he already knew that was true. Vaughn became still and stared off into the distance for a long time. I could feel him sorting through different thoughts to find what he was looking for. Suddenly, he popped out of contemplation and grabbed his iPad to type a message. "Then I can feel good about myself right now, and for no reason except I exist!"

"That's it! How does that feel?" I asked.

"I'm elated and I feel free," he replied. "How do I hold onto this?"

"You don't need to hold on to anything. It's a moment by moment choice that you get to make. As the saying goes, 'The Goddess always says yes!' So, you can choose to try to force and control your life, or you can surrender completely beyond your desire to control life.

"When you surrender your sense of separateness, you experience yourself as part of the deep, rich flow of mysterious complexity of Creation. This is not something your linear mind can ever understand, but it is something you can experience. The resonances of Creation itself are so vast and profound that they create your life effortlessly, elegantly and gracefully.

"The linear mind most definitely does not agree with or understand this perspective," I continued, trying to give him a sense of how things actually work despite appearances to the contrary. "Our primitive brain is not the seat of our consciousness

The Beautiful Language of the Heart

even though it's quite sure that it is. It wants to understand and control everything.

"This mental survival-oriented part of us is only one small element within our larger consciousness. Most people have lived exclusively within the mind's limited perspectives and believe that it's the only thing that's real. While we can't force the limited part of us to change its point of view, we can become aware that there's much more to our consciousness. Then we can explore more expansive parts of ourselves.

"We have parts of our brain, and also our consciousness itself, that transcend our survival hardwiring. In learning to feel the difference, we can live from the relaxed calm of that lighter and freer perspective.

"When we include our primitive brain as only a very small part of who we are, and not as the whole, our consciousness expands. As we see its limited perspectives for what they are, which is our old flat consciousness, we become less and less seduced by its fear-based stories.

"Vaughn, would you like to experience this?" He nodded excitedly.

"First, can you hear those voices in your head that try to convince you that you are not already whole, valued and loved? What are those voices saying and how do they feel in your body?"

"They say there's something wrong with me. It's dark, depressing, and despairing," he typed with a heavy sigh.

"What if those voices are telling you the opposite of what's true about you?" I suggested. "What if your inner light is actually stronger than those negative beliefs that are trying to seduce you to agree with their point of view?"

"I know you're right and I would like to feel that," he replied.

"Are you confident that your light is stronger?" I inquired.

"I'm confident until I am not," was his inimitable reply. Ryan and I glanced at each other, enjoying the brilliant way Vaughn expressed profound truth.

"Next time you lose your confidence, remember that you aren't separate from your inner source of light. You're already full of that light. In fact, you are the light itself!"

*You already are
more magnificent
and full of light
than you can ever
imagine!*

"Then why do I lose my confidence and not feel that I am full of light? What can I do about that?" He sincerely wanted to know.

"What if you were to start from the premise that you are not empty, nor are you separate from the light. You are already completely full of your inner source of light. How would you feel if you were already infinitely appreciated, approved of, valued, loved, cherished, and adored by the light and all of Creation? It's already true, even when you don't let yourself feel it.

"It's much more empowering to experience the truth of who you already are than to put energy into seeking, needing, and wanting or denying. Why not live from the potency of the light that you already are, rather than from the misperception that you are not that? The more you open into your inner source of light, the more free and joyous you become."

The Beautiful Language of the Heart

*One of the greatest gifts
we get to receive in life
is the experience of
being the light
itself.*

"Vaughn, would you like to try that now?" He was always eager for new experiences. "Those negative voices are there, but you don't need to get rid of them, fight with them, or follow them down the rabbit hole. While we can't trust the content of our fear-based stories, we can trust the flow of our limitless consciousness.

"To feel this, let's start by taking a few gentle breaths and let time slow down. Let's do this together a few times. Now open more space in your body. Notice how your energy deepens and expands. Can you also feel the presence of the heaviness of those negative beliefs? You don't need to fix or get rid of them. Just hold yourself in love and compassion for having the heavy fear-based stories. It's not your fault they are there. We all have them in different colors, shapes and sizes.

"What happens when you accept that those voices are there at this moment? You don't have to agree with them or even like them. You can wish they weren't there and still include them because they are there. Then at the same time also feel that who you are is so far greater. That means realizing that those voices are there, and at the same time you are a limitless being whose heart is vast enough to hold those limited voices. Round.

"Being real, which means being authentic, doesn't mean being perfect or resolving the fear stories of our primitive brain. We don't need to replace their negative stories with positive ones.

Anamika

That's like putting whipped cream on worms."

Our authentic self
is
beyond all stories.
Who we are
is
an experience.

"Nothing is wrong with any part of us, and we can hold every bit as precious. We don't even have to work hard to get somewhere because there's nowhere to get. There isn't a place where we are finally perfect and finished."

We are already whole
even while
becoming
more.
We are lacking nothing.
We are far greater
than we can
possibly imagine.
In our limitlessness
"I" is much too small a word.
"We"
which includes
"I"
is who we are.

The Beautiful Language of the Heart

As Vaughn expanded into his limitless self, the room filled with gorgeous light. Ryan was sitting next to Vaughn and felt it strongly too. We closed our eyes to soak in its radiance, and bask in the warmth of its rays. In that moment, Vaughn realized that nothing more was needed because he was filled with what he longed to feel, and so much more than he could have imagined.

The flow of these luminous energies rewrites our core programming as it catalyzes change in us. We don't ever need to stay stuck because we have the choice to open into these energies whenever we want. What keeps us feeling stuck comes from the greatest illusion humans have. The illusion is that we are separate from, and not one with, the light of Creation itself. Flat. Separation is an illusion. We are completely connected and part of All That Is, so we can never actually be separate. Round.

"Sometimes I feel like a victim of my life, but what you're telling me is very empowering," he admitted.

"Feeling like a victim comes from the flat perspective that life is happening to you, and you have no choice about it. It appears that the world is outside of us and separate from us, but this is not so. Our life, and what we call reality are created from our inner beliefs and their resonances of energy. Our mind can't understand this because it seems like it's the opposite way around. The mind also thinks we have no choice about life. But, we are always free to choose new perspectives.

"As you've already experienced, when you change your perspective it changes the way you feel. This new embodied energy changes not only our experience of reality, but changes our outer reality itself. These new resonances alter what we feel, what we're able to perceive, and how we relate to all that exists, or All That Is.

Anamika

"Our inner resonances create our outer reality from the inside out which means that our outer life is an expression of our inner beliefs and resonances. When we change our perspectives and our inner resonances, our outer life follows suit. So, if you don't like something that's happening in your life, change your inner perspectives and your outer life will follow. This is absolutely impossible for the linear mind to understand, because it looks like it's the other way around."

Nothing changes until we do.
Everything changes when we do.

The deeply ingrained perception that we are separate and just an individual small "I" renders us powerless, victimized and stuck. We are hardwired with this misperception, which makes it feel so real. But when we are willing to also include the limitless part of us, so that we are both the smaller and the larger parts, it opens us to new perceptions and experiences of life and reality.

Our third-dimensional, little "I" self isn't bad or wrong. It's just extraordinarily limited and only applies to a tiny slice of space/time. When we believe that third-dimensional reality is all that exists, we then extrapolate and say that its limited perspective applies to everything, everywhere and always.

Since we can't see more than third-dimensional reality with our common senses, many say it doesn't exist. But multidimensional reality does exist and is infinitely more vast and rich. We can perceive it with our uncommon senses that let us see, hear, and touch limitless realms of energy.

"Is this why I remember so many past lives? I seem to operate differently than many other people," he typed.

"Yes! Our consciousness itself exists within and also beyond time and space. You operate differently because you have access to multidimensional aspects of your consciousness outside of time and space. Many people don't yet have access to that, so they think it doesn't exist. Without that conscious awareness, it looks like life is only a linear cause and effect reality.

"Quantum physics has described the existence of energy behaving in a non-linear fashion, like both a wave and a particle, for example. In addition, the mere act of indirectly observing the atomic realm changes the outcome of its interactions. Thus, everything is interconnected and always changing, which we can experience for ourselves when we open multidimensionally beyond the space-time continuum."

Vaughn and I were both excited about his revelations. Since he loved practicing what he learned, he came to our next session wanting to know how to reconcile his third-dimensional and multidimensional selves.

"Being authentic includes your little 'I' and your limitless self. When you are in touch with your authentic self, which includes all of who you are, you have far greater impact than you can imagine."

The notion of having impact moved him so deeply that he revealed his true passion. "What I really want to do is share what I've learned in order to help people. I want to make a difference."

"There's your beautiful heart speaking again, Vaughn. The more you come from your heart, the more impact you have; it grows exponentially."

Vaughn's face became full of hope. I could see how deeply he cared about connecting with others and touching their lives, so I wanted to help him have greater access to his authentic self.

"To live an extraordinary life requires including both our finite three- dimensional and our limitless multidimensional nature. They are both part of our authentic self. It's and/and. We can appreciate each for what it is, without trying to force one to be the other. In accepting and including both, they ultimately support each other and something completely new emerges that is greater than the sum of the parts. That's your authentic self, born of the paradox of *and*.

"When we include all of who we are with love and compassion, from the most limited to the most limitless, we are continually integrating and enlightening. This process goes on forever and is quite fun when our relationship with All That Is becomes a conscious co-creation. All of the different parts of us cooperate in creating reality instantaneously, in each moment."

I am me
and
one with All That Is
continuously integrating and enlightening
becoming more of
who I am
and
more of
who we are
and
more
and…

The Beautiful Language of the Heart

Is this enlightenment? No. There isn't a place or achievement called enlightenment. There is continuous enlightening, unfolding, and becoming. We never arrive, and it never stops.

Enlightening
goes
on
forever
and
so
do
we.

Through deep acceptance of All as it is, we can see the aliveness in all things. Everything doesn't have the same consciousness, but everything has aliveness. Life itself is alive. It's a great gift and within its depths is magic.

Magic isn't linear or logical, and it doesn't follow our ideas about how it should work. Our ideas try to fit magic into a cause and effect reality but it doesn't work that way. When operating at its highest levels, it leaves no evidence of its presence. In leaving no trace, magic can change our life instantaneously, as if "by magic."

The energy which creates, giving birth to new life, is so much bigger than we are. When we come into harmony with it, we stop trying to boss it around, fix it, or contain it. Instead, we get to experience the awe-inspiring mystery of being part of Creation creating anew.

Creation has its own brilliant intelligence and although we

think we're the ones who know it all, we actually don't. Moreover, we don't need to know how it works, but rather be willing to experience it.

Pause and feel
the awe
and
miracle
of your own existence.

The multidimensionality of Creation is like a magnificent kaleidoscope that keeps moving and changing. Rather than trying to control it, micromanage it, or freeze it in place, we get to enjoy and explore it. Those are completely different paradigms. Flat to round. Trying to control it would be like trying to control the ocean.

We've heard the phrase, "We create our own reality." Many people confuse this to mean, "I get to control my reality." However, control is a very different process than being in harmony with, and part of Creation creating anew.

When we think of life as a series of challenges we have to overcome, we struggle. When we open to the perspective that life itself wants to support us, and does support us, we relax into a resonance field of infinite abundance. From there, we don't need to make life happen. Instead, we get to receive it abundantly and effortlessly.

Imagine life without struggle
delighting in how it moves
instead of trying
to control how it unfolds.

The Beautiful Language of the Heart

Within this perspective, we are in harmony with All That Is, because we're already one with it. As we embrace this round consciousness, we see with new eyes and are able to perceive what we couldn't see before.

New creation is like the sun exploding inside of us. It's full of substance, warmth, movement, and light expanding in all directions simultaneously. It's like an internal fusion reactor that produces a net gain of new vitality and aliveness that are life-giving. We are part of birthing, rather than controlling reality.

*More important than
who or what
we're becoming
is
that
we're becoming.
This is our true artistry.*

Real artists don't know ahead of time what they're creating. They stand with delight in the convergence of the unfolding and enfolding of All That Is. The confluence of All That Is converging as a singular point of space, time and consciousness miraculously is a "big bang" which creates the "matter" that is us. We are not solid matter but a series of big bangs flashing so quickly, it's unfathomable.

*Each exquisite moment of connection
with All That Is
changes our lives forever.*

Anamika

We become an artist of life itself
birthing Creation together.

Our splendid uniqueness
in concert with All That Is
is a mutually thrilling
love affair.
A romance
intensely alive
utterly sensual
sublimely erotic
passionate
fulfilling.
A dance of
unparalleled pleasure
luscious communing
inexpressibly joyous entwining.

Never-ending
eternally
more
rich
luminous
intense
intimate.
Exquisite
beyond delicious.

For every truth we discover, there will always be a deeper one.

The Beautiful Language of the Heart

For every wonder we experience, there will always be a more astonishing one. No matter what octave of peace and joy we reach, there's always more to be explored.

When we go far enough into this new consciousness, we receive and create spontaneously from our heart's truest desires, which are feelings, not things. We are one with All That Is exploring All That Is in an infinite variety of ways.

We're being invited to experience our authentic self in conscious co-creation with All That Is. Together, we co-create ourselves and reality instantaneously in each moment.

It's where evolution
is
inviting us
to go.

"So, my dearest Vaughn, to live an extraordinary life, here's the magic formula:"

Show up and be present
let go of everything you've ever believed
open to new perspectives
receive from the magic and mystery of life
celebrate!

Vaughn lit up immediately and was beaming his brilliant light.

"I have a question for you, Vaughn. How do you go there so effortlessly?"

"I focus on the feeling of what you're saying and it lightens and warms my true inner self."

As Ryan and I exchanged a look of delight as Vaughn displayed his wisdom yet again, Vaughn jumped up from his chair. This time it wasn't to run out of the room. Instead, he took his place in the center of the room and began to twirl and twirl and twirl and twirl and twirl, doing his happy dance.

Living joyously

in

the present

celebrating the never-ending

exhilaration

elation

and

thrill

of our

miraculous existence.

A huge smile covered his face and rays of joy were radiating from his whole being. "That's it, Vaughn, you've got it! You're speaking the beautiful language of the heart!"

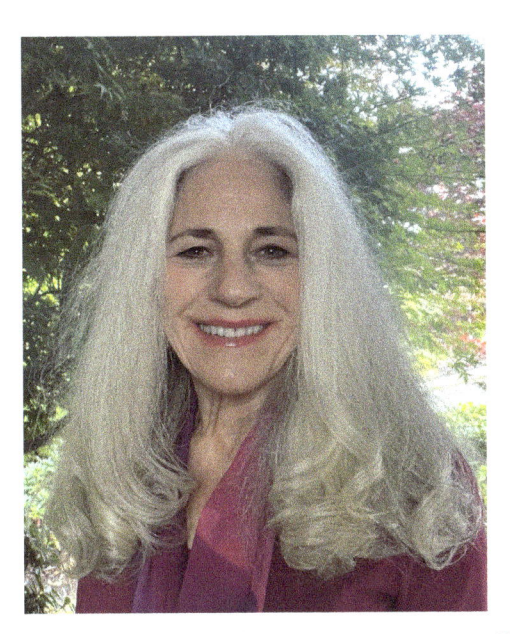

About the Author

Anamika has been exploring the limitless multidimensionality of reality, existence, and human consciousness for over forty-five years. She shares her experiences through private sessions, workshops, online seminars and authored *The Beautiful Language of the Heart* book and companion documentary, *and...*, *Loving Now*, *Love in Fur Coats*, and *French Lessons in Love*. https://anamika.com/beautiful-language-heart.

With a B.A. in Psychology from Wellesley College, a Ph.D. from Columbia Pacific University, she also graduated from The Barbara Brennan School of Healing. Her background includes spiritual metaphysics, psychology, energy healing, holistic health, music, dance, and French. She lives with her partner in Washington, USA and loves hiking with her Afghan Hound, Zig. anamika.com.

Introducing The Beautiful Language of the Heart Documentary

When I first began to work with Vaughn in 2020, I was deeply moved by the gems of wisdom, understanding, and transformation that were occurring in our Zoom sessions. When I proposed the idea of taping the sessions, Vaughn and his parents agreed, hoping that his experiences of healing and becoming more of his real self would help others too.

After taping our weekly sessions for two years, I compiled the material into a two-part documentary depicting the evolution of finding oneself. The documentary was launched in 2022 and received outstanding reviews. Vaughn attended some of the showings and got to see how touching and empowering his story was to other people, and the many ways in which his journey was universal and applicable to everyone.

When Sarah Ferguson watched the documentary, she let me know that she had gained so much from it personally. When she

The Beautiful Language of the Heart

suggested that it could give courage and hope to people globally, she inspired me to make his story even more widely available by writing this book.

The Beautiful Language of the Heart Documentary is available to view, free of charge, at https://anamika.com/beautiful-language-heart.